First-Time Mum Pregnancy Handbook

An Expectant Mother's Week-By-Week Guide on What to Expect During Pregnancy

Watson R. Ward

Copyright ©

Watson R. Ward

© 2024 USA

Gratitude

Thank you from the bottom of my heart for choosing to embark on this incredible journey with me by your side.

I am truly honored that you've picked up this First-Time Mum Pregnancy Handbook to be a part of your pregnancy adventure.

Pregnancy is a time filled with excitement, wonder, and a fair share of uncertainties. My hope is that this book brings you comfort, knowledge, and a sense of companionship as you navigate these precious months.

Every page was written with you in mind, aiming to offer the support and encouragement you deserve.

I want you to know that you are not alone. There are countless mothers-to-be who are feeling exactly what you're feeling, and we're all in this together.

Whether you're experiencing joy, anxiety, or a mix of both, this book is here to be your friend, your guide, and your source of reassurance.

Thank you for allowing me to be a part of your special journey. Your trust and support mean the world to me.

Wishing you a beautiful pregnancy filled with love, health, and unforgettable moments.

Table of Contents

Introduction

Hello, beautiful mum-to-be!

First of all, congratulations! Finding out that you're pregnant is one of the most exciting and transformative moments in life.

Whether you've been planning for this or it came as a surprise, you're about to embark on a journey filled with wonder, joy, and a fair share of challenges. This book is here to walk beside you every step of the way.

Becoming a mother for the first time can feel overwhelming. There's so much to learn, so many decisions to make, and a whirlwind of emotions to navigate.

That's where this handbook comes in. Think of it as your trusty companion, a friendly guide who's here to offer advice, share knowledge, and provide a comforting word when you need it most.

Inside these pages, you'll find practical tips, heartfelt encouragement, and plenty of information to help you feel prepared and empowered. From the moment you find out you're pregnant to those precious first days with your newborn, this book covers it all.

But more than just a guide, it's a conversation between friends – because you deserve to feel supported and understood during this incredible time.

How to Use This Handbook

Each chapter of this book is designed to address the different stages and aspects of your pregnancy.

Whether you're looking for advice on dealing with morning sickness, wondering how to set up the perfect nursery, or curious about what labor will really be like, you'll find it all here.

You don't have to read it cover to cover – feel free to jump to the sections that speak to you at the moment.

Remember, every pregnancy is unique. What works for one person might not work for another, and that's okay.

This book is filled with a variety of tips and suggestions so you can find what fits best for you and your baby. Trust your instincts and give yourself grace – you are doing an amazing job!

Let's Get Started

I'm so excited to share this journey with you. Pregnancy is a time of profound change, but also a time of incredible growth and love.

As you read through this handbook, know that you are part of a community of mothers who are here to support you. You are not alone.

So, grab a cozy blanket, make yourself a cup of tea, and let's dive in. Here's to a wonderful journey ahead!

Finding Out You're Pregnant

Discovering that you're pregnant is a moment you'll never forget. Whether you had an inkling that something was different or it came as a total surprise, that positive pregnancy test is a life-changing event.

Let's take a moment to breathe, smile, and celebrate this incredible news!

The Moment of Truth

Picture this: It's early morning, and you're holding that little stick with bated breath. You might be alone, or perhaps your partner is anxiously waiting beside you.

Then, like magic, those two little lines or the word "pregnant" appears. Your heart skips a beat, your eyes widen, and emotions start swirling – excitement, joy, disbelief, maybe even a touch of fear. All of these feelings are completely normal and natural.

Take a deep breath. This is real. You're going to be a mum!

Processing the News

After the initial shock, it's time to let the news sink in. You might find yourself laughing, crying, or sitting in stunned silence.

Give yourself permission to feel whatever comes naturally. There's no right or wrong way to react.

If your partner is with you, share this beautiful moment together. Hug, cry, laugh, and talk about the future.

If you're on your own, consider calling a close friend or family member to share your joy. No matter what, remember that you have support around you.

First Steps Forward

Now that the big news is out in the open, there are a few important steps to take:

Confirm with a Healthcare Provider: Schedule an appointment with your doctor or midwife to confirm your pregnancy. They'll likely do a blood test and possibly an early ultrasound to ensure everything is on track.

Start Prenatal Vitamins: If you haven't already, start taking prenatal vitamins with folic acid. These are crucial for your baby's early development.

Celebrate! This is a moment worth celebrating. Whether it's a quiet evening with your partner, a small gathering with close friends, or simply a solo dance party in your living room, do something special to mark this new chapter.

Telling Your Partner and Loved Ones

Sharing the news with your partner and loved ones can be one of the most joyous parts of this experience. If you haven't told your partner yet, think about how you'd like to share the news. Some people go for a sweet surprise, like a special gift or card, while others prefer a direct and heartfelt conversation.

When it comes to telling family and friends, you have a few weeks to decide how and when. Some people prefer to wait until after the first trimester when the risk of miscarriage decreases, while others can't wait to shout it from the rooftops. Do what feels right for you.

Embracing the Journey Ahead

As the news settles in, allow yourself to start dreaming about the future. Picture holding your baby for the first time, imagine their tiny fingers and toes, and think about all the wonderful moments to come.

Remember, this is just the beginning of an incredible journey. There will be ups and downs, surprises, and challenges, but through it all, you are embarking on one of life's most amazing adventures. You've got this, and you're not alone.

First Things First: What to Do Right Away

Finding out you're pregnant is a moment of pure magic, but it can also feel a bit overwhelming. With so many thoughts racing through your mind, it's important to take a few practical steps to set the stage for a healthy and happy pregnancy. Let's break it down together, step by step.

Confirm Your Pregnancy

Your at-home pregnancy test is a good indicator, but it's important to confirm the news with a healthcare provider.

Schedule an appointment with your doctor or midwife as soon as possible. They'll perform a blood test or an early ultrasound to confirm your pregnancy and give you an estimated due date.

This initial visit is also a great time to ask any burning questions you have.

Start Taking Prenatal Vitamins

If you haven't already, now is the time to start taking prenatal vitamins. These vitamins are specially formulated to support your baby's development and your own health.

Look for a vitamin that includes folic acid, iron, calcium, and DHA. Folic acid is especially important in the early weeks to help prevent neural tube defects.

Evaluate Your Lifestyle

This is a good time to take a look at your lifestyle and make any necessary adjustments to ensure a healthy pregnancy:

Nutrition: Start incorporating a variety of fruits, vegetables, whole grains, and lean proteins into your diet. Try to limit processed foods, caffeine, and sugary drinks.

Exercise: Staying active is great for both you and your baby. Aim for moderate exercise like walking, swimming, or prenatal yoga. Always check with your healthcare provider before starting any new workout routine.

Avoid Harmful Substances: Say goodbye to alcohol, smoking, and recreational drugs. If you need help quitting, talk to your healthcare provider for resources and support.

Schedule Your First Prenatal Visit

Your first prenatal visit will likely be around 8 to 10 weeks into your pregnancy. During this visit, your healthcare provider will take a detailed medical history, perform a physical exam, and run some routine tests. They'll also discuss your prenatal care plan and answer any questions you might have.

Learn About Your Insurance and Maternity Leave

Take some time to understand your health insurance coverage and what's included for prenatal care, labor, and delivery. Also, if you're working, find out about your company's maternity leave policy.

Knowing your options early on can help you plan better for the months ahead.

Start a Pregnancy Journal

Keeping a pregnancy journal can be a wonderful way to document this special time. Write down your feelings, thoughts, and any milestones or symptoms you experience.

This journal will not only be a cherished keepsake but can also help you track your pregnancy progress and prepare for discussions with your healthcare provider.

Begin Reading and Researching

There's a lot to learn about pregnancy, childbirth, and parenting. Start reading reputable books, articles, and websites to educate yourself about what to expect. Just remember, every pregnancy is unique, so take in the information that feels right for you and your situation.

Join a Support Group

Connecting with other expecting mums can be incredibly reassuring and helpful. Look for local or online pregnancy support groups where you can share experiences, ask questions, and receive encouragement from others who are going through the same journey.

Taking It One Step at a Time

It's easy to feel like you need to do everything all at once, but remember, pregnancy is a marathon, not a sprint. Take it one step at a time and be kind to yourself.

Each small step you take is a step toward a healthy, happy pregnancy for you and your baby.

Your First Trimester (Weeks 1-12)

What to Expect: Physical and Emotional Changes

Welcome to the rollercoaster of pregnancy! The first trimester is a time of incredible transformation, both physically and emotionally.

Your body is working hard to support your growing baby, and with that comes a variety of changes. Let's dive into what you can expect and how to navigate these new experiences.

Physical Changes

Morning Sickness: Despite the name, morning sickness can strike at any time of the day. Nausea and vomiting are common and usually begin around the sixth week of pregnancy. Try eating small, frequent meals and keeping snacks like crackers or ginger handy. Stay hydrated and rest as much as you can.

Breast Tenderness: Hormonal changes can make your breasts feel swollen, tender, and sensitive. A good supportive bra can make a world of difference.

Fatigue: Growing a baby is hard work! It's normal to feel unusually tired. Listen to your body and get plenty of rest. Nap when you can and don't hesitate to ask for help with daily tasks.

Frequent Urination: Your body produces more blood during pregnancy, which leads to extra fluid being processed by your kidneys. This can result in more trips to the bathroom. Stay hydrated but try to limit fluids before bedtime.

Food Cravings and Aversions: You might find yourself craving certain foods and being turned off by others. This is completely normal. Try to maintain a balanced diet but don't be too hard on yourself if you indulge in your cravings occasionally.

Bloating and Constipation: Hormonal changes can slow down your digestive system, leading to bloating and constipation. Drink plenty of water, eat fiber-rich foods, and stay active to help keep things moving.

Spotting and Cramping: Light spotting and mild cramping can occur as the fertilized egg implants itself into the lining of your uterus. If the spotting is heavy or accompanied by severe pain, contact your healthcare provider.

Emotional Changes

Mood Swings: Hormones are surging, and it's natural to experience mood swings. You might feel ecstatic one moment and weepy the next. Be kind to yourself and talk to someone you trust about your feelings.

Anxiety and Worry: It's normal to worry about your baby's health, your changing body, and the future. Remember, it's okay to have these feelings. Discuss any concerns with your healthcare provider and lean on your support network.

Joy and Excitement: Amidst the challenges, there will be moments of pure joy and excitement. Embrace these feelings and allow yourself to dream about your baby and the future.

Forgetfulness: "Pregnancy brain" is a real thing! Hormonal changes and fatigue can make you feel forgetful or scattered. Keep a notepad or use your phone to jot down reminders and important dates.

Embrace the Journey

Remember, every pregnancy is unique. Some days will be easier than others, but each day brings you closer to meeting your little one.

Celebrate the small victories, and be gentle with yourself through the challenges. You are doing an amazing job, and your body is performing a miraculous task.

Coping with Morning Sickness and Fatigue

The first trimester can be a bit of a whirlwind, with your body adjusting to the amazing changes happening inside.

Two of the most common (and often challenging) symptoms you might face are morning sickness and fatigue.

But don't worry – you're not alone, and there are plenty of ways to manage these feelings. Let's dive into some tips and tricks to help you cope.

Morning Sickness: It's Not Just for Mornings

Morning sickness can actually strike at any time of day, and for some mums-to-be, it can be quite relentless.

Here's how to navigate those queasy moments:

Eat Small, Frequent Meals: Keeping your stomach from becoming too empty or too full can help stabilize your blood sugar levels and reduce nausea. Aim for small, frequent meals throughout the day rather than three large ones.

Snack Smart: Keep easy-to-digest snacks on hand, such as crackers, plain toast, or pretzels. Foods high in protein, like nuts or cheese, can also help. Ginger is known for its anti-nausea properties, so try ginger tea, ginger ale, or ginger candies.

Stay Hydrated: Sip on water, herbal teas, or electrolyte drinks throughout the day. If plain water isn't appealing, try adding a slice of lemon or a splash of juice. Cold, clear liquids might be easier to tolerate.

Avoid Triggers: Pay attention to what sets off your nausea. Common triggers include certain smells, spicy foods, and greasy or heavy meals. Once you identify your triggers, do your best to avoid them.

Rest and Relax: Stress and fatigue can worsen nausea, so make sure you're getting plenty of rest.

Practice relaxation techniques like deep breathing, meditation, or gentle yoga.

Try Acupressure: Acupressure wristbands, often used for motion sickness, can sometimes help alleviate nausea. They're available at most pharmacies and are easy to use.

Talk to Your Healthcare Provider: If your morning sickness is severe or you're unable to keep anything down, it's important to talk to your healthcare provider.

They might recommend vitamin B6 supplements or other medications to help manage your symptoms.

Fatigue: Rest When You Can

Feeling extra tired is completely normal during the first trimester. Your body is working overtime to support your baby's development, so it's important to listen to your body and rest when needed:

Nap When Possible: If your schedule allows, take short naps during the day. Even a 20-30 minute nap can help recharge your energy levels.

Prioritize Sleep: Aim for 7-9 hours of sleep each night. Create a calming bedtime routine to help you wind down – think warm baths, reading a book, or listening to soothing music.

Stay Active: While it might seem counterintuitive, gentle exercise can actually boost your energy levels. Activities like walking, swimming, or prenatal yoga can help you feel more awake and invigorated.

Eat Nutrient-Rich Foods: A balanced diet can help combat fatigue. Focus on foods rich in iron (like leafy greens and lean meats), protein, and complex carbohydrates. Avoid too much sugar and caffeine, as they can lead to energy crashes.

Stay Hydrated: Dehydration can contribute to feelings of fatigue, so make sure you're drinking enough fluids throughout the day.

Ask for Help: Don't be afraid to ask for help with household chores or other responsibilities. Friends and family are often more than willing to lend a hand, especially when they know you're expecting.

Manage Stress: High stress levels can drain your energy. Find healthy ways to manage stress, whether it's through mindfulness practices, talking to a friend, or spending time on a hobby you enjoy.

Morning sickness and fatigue are often most intense during the first trimester and typically improve as you enter the second trimester.

Be patient with yourself and give your body the rest and nourishment it needs. Every pregnancy is unique, so find what works best for you and take it one day at a time.

Nutrition and Diet: Eating for Two

Nutrition and Diet: Eating for Two

Eating for two doesn't mean doubling your portions, but it does mean being mindful of what you're putting into your body.

Your diet plays a crucial role in your baby's development and your own health. Let's explore some practical tips to help you nourish both yourself and your growing baby.

Balanced Diet Basics

Your body needs a variety of nutrients to support a healthy pregnancy.

Here are the key components of a balanced diet:

Proteins: Essential for your baby's growth and development. Good sources include lean meats, poultry, fish, eggs, beans, nuts, and seeds.

Fruits and Vegetables: Packed with vitamins, minerals, and fiber. Aim for a colorful variety to ensure you're getting a range of nutrients.

Whole Grains: Provide energy and important nutrients like fiber, iron, and B vitamins. Choose whole grains like brown rice, whole wheat bread, quinoa, and oats.

Dairy: Important for calcium and vitamin D. Include milk, cheese, yogurt, or fortified plant-based alternatives like almond or soy milk.

Healthy Fats: Essential for brain development. Include sources like avocados, nuts, seeds, olive oil, and fatty fish like salmon (but limit high-mercury fish).

Key Nutrients for Pregnancy

Certain nutrients are particularly important during pregnancy:

Folic Acid: Crucial for preventing neural tube defects. Found in leafy greens, citrus fruits, beans, and fortified cereals. Your prenatal vitamin should also contain folic acid.

Iron: Supports the increased blood volume and helps prevent anemia. Found in lean meats, spinach, lentils, and iron-fortified cereals.

Pair iron-rich foods with vitamin C-rich foods (like oranges or bell peppers) to enhance absorption.

Calcium: Important for your baby's bone development. Found in dairy products, fortified plant-based milks, leafy greens, and almonds.

Vitamin D: Helps with calcium absorption and bone health. Found in fatty fish, fortified milk, and sunlight exposure. Your healthcare provider might recommend a supplement if needed.

Omega-3 Fatty Acids: Essential for brain development. Found in fatty fish, flaxseeds, chia seeds, and walnuts.

Eating Tips for a Healthy Pregnancy

Eat Small, Frequent Meals: This can help manage nausea and keep your energy levels stable. Aim for three main meals and two to three healthy snacks each day.

Stay Hydrated: Drink plenty of water throughout the day. Aim for at least eight glasses, more if you're active. Herbal teas and soups can also contribute to your fluid intake.

Limit Caffeine: Keep caffeine intake to 200 mg per day, which is about one 12-ounce cup of coffee. Remember, caffeine is also found in tea, chocolate, and some soft drinks.

Avoid Certain Foods: Steer clear of raw or undercooked seafood, eggs, and meats; unpasteurized dairy products; and high-mercury fish like shark, swordfish, and king mackerel.

Also, avoid deli meats and hot dogs unless they're heated to steaming hot.

Watch Out for Food Safety: Practice good food hygiene by washing fruits and vegetables thoroughly, cooking meats to safe temperatures, and avoiding cross-contamination in the kitchen.

Listen to Your Body: Cravings and aversions are normal. It's okay to indulge occasionally, but try to balance treats with nutrient-dense foods.

If you're feeling full quickly, focus on nutrient-rich snacks like yogurt with fruit, a handful of nuts, or a smoothie.

Dealing with Common Issues

Nausea: If morning sickness is making it hard to eat, try bland, easy-to-digest foods like crackers, plain toast, or bananas. Ginger and peppermint teas can also help settle your stomach.

Heartburn: Avoid spicy, fatty, or acidic foods that can trigger heartburn. Eat smaller meals and avoid lying down immediately after eating.

Constipation: Increase your fiber intake with fruits, vegetables, whole grains, and legumes. Drink plenty of water and stay active to keep things moving.

Enjoying Your Food

Pregnancy is a wonderful time to explore new foods and recipes. Try to make mealtime enjoyable and stress-free.

Experiment with healthy, delicious recipes that satisfy your cravings and nourish your body. Remember, it's not just about eating the right foods, but also about enjoying the journey.

You're Nourishing a New Life

Every bite you take is a step toward nurturing your baby and yourself. Embrace this opportunity to build healthy habits that will benefit you both.

Listen to your body, make thoughtful choices, and don't be too hard on yourself if things don't go perfectly every day. You're doing an amazing job!

Your Second Trimester (Weeks 13-26)

The Honeymoon Phase: Feeling Better and Energy Boost

Congratulations, you've made it to the second trimester! This period is often referred to as the "honeymoon phase" of pregnancy – a time when many mums-to-be start to feel more energetic and comfortable.

Let's dive into what you can expect during this exciting phase and how to make the most of it.

Feeling Better: A Welcome Relief

For many women, the second trimester brings a welcome relief from some of the early pregnancy symptoms:

Reduced Nausea: Morning sickness often subsides, allowing you to enjoy your meals again. Embrace this change and focus on maintaining a balanced diet to support your growing baby.

Increased Energy: You might find that your energy levels start to pick up, making you feel more like yourself again. This is a great time to get back to activities you enjoy and prepare for the months ahead.

Emotional Stability: Hormonal fluctuations often stabilize, leading to a more balanced mood. You might feel more emotionally steady and able to enjoy your pregnancy more fully.

Planning and Preparing

The second trimester is an ideal time to start planning and preparing for your baby's arrival:

Start Your Registry: With your energy levels up, now is a great time to start your baby registry. Research the items you'll need and make a list of must-haves and nice-to-haves.

Prepare the Nursery: Begin setting up your baby's nursery. Whether it's painting the walls, assembling furniture, or organizing baby clothes, this is a fun and productive way to use your energy.

Take a Babymoon: If you're feeling up to it, consider taking a babymoon – a relaxing getaway before your baby arrives. Choose a destination where you can unwind and enjoy some quality time with your partner.

Educate Yourself: Use this time to read up on childbirth and parenting. Attend prenatal classes, read books, and join online forums to connect with other expecting mums.

Connecting with Your Baby

As your baby grows, you'll start to feel those first fluttering movements, known as quickening. This is an exciting milestone that helps you feel more connected to your baby:

Bonding Time: Talk to your baby, play music, and gently rub your belly. These small gestures can help strengthen the bond between you and your little one.

Keep a Journal: Document your feelings, thoughts, and experiences in a pregnancy journal. This is a wonderful way to reflect on your journey and create lasting memories.

Prenatal Appointments: Continue attending your prenatal appointments to monitor your baby's development and address any questions or concerns you might have.

Enjoy the Ride

The second trimester is often the most enjoyable phase of pregnancy, so take advantage of it! Embrace the positive changes and make time for activities that bring you joy and relaxation. Remember to take care of yourself and celebrate the small victories along the way.

You're doing an amazing job, and your baby is growing stronger every day. Enjoy this special time and the beautiful journey of pregnancy.

Baby's Development: What's Happening Inside

As you journey through your pregnancy, it's incredible to think about the miraculous changes happening inside your body.

During the second trimester, your baby grows and develops at a rapid pace, transforming from a tiny embryo into a recognizable little human.

Let's explore the fascinating journey of your baby's development during this stage.

Weeks 13-16: Growth Spurts and Movement

By the end of the first trimester, your baby is about the size of a peach. As you enter the second trimester:

Growth Spurt: Your baby undergoes a growth spurt, doubling in size by week 14. They now have distinct facial features, tiny fingernails, and even tooth buds beneath their gums.

Movement: You may start to feel those first flutters of movement, known as quickening. At first, it may feel like butterflies or gentle taps. These movements will become more pronounced as your baby grows stronger.

Organs and Systems: Internal organs continue to develop and mature. The kidneys begin to produce urine, and the intestines start to move into their proper place in the abdomen.

Weeks 17-20: Developing Senses and Vernix

As your baby reaches the halfway point of gestation:

Senses: Your baby's senses are developing. They can now hear sounds from the outside world, including your voice and heartbeat. Their eyes are formed but remain closed.

Vernix Caseosa: A waxy coating called vernix caseosa begins to cover your baby's skin. This protective layer helps regulate their body temperature and protects their delicate skin from the amniotic fluid.

Growth Milestones: Your baby is growing rapidly, and you might have a mid-pregnancy ultrasound (around week 20) to check their growth and anatomy. This is often when you can find out the sex of your baby if you choose to.

Weeks 21-26: Rapid Brain Development

In the later weeks of the second trimester:

Brain Development: Your baby's brain undergoes significant growth and development. They start forming billions of neurons and developing the structures that will control their movements, senses, and thoughts.

Breathing Practice: Your baby begins practicing breathing movements. While they're surrounded by amniotic fluid and don't breathe air, these practice breaths help develop their respiratory muscles.

Eyesight: Eyelids, which have been fused shut, begin to open, and your baby's eyesight continues to develop. They can perceive light filtering through your belly, although their vision is still very basic.

Bonding with Your Baby

Feeling connected to your growing baby is a beautiful part of pregnancy:

Talking and Singing: Your baby can hear your voice and may even respond to familiar sounds. Take time to talk, sing, and read to your baby. This helps strengthen your bond and promotes their early brain development.

Touching Your Belly: Gently touching and rubbing your belly can reassure your baby and create a comforting connection between the two of you.

Ultrasound Moments: Seeing your baby during ultrasounds can be incredibly special. Take these opportunities to marvel at their growth and share the excitement with your partner and loved ones.

Your Baby, Your Journey

Every pregnancy is unique, and your baby is developing at their own pace. Trust that your body knows how to nurture and support this incredible process. As you continue on this journey, take time to appreciate the wonder of new life growing inside you.

Stay connected with your healthcare provider for regular check-ups and enjoy the anticipation of meeting your little one. You're doing an amazing job nurturing your baby's growth and well-being.

Maternity Fashion: Comfort and Style Tips

Pregnancy is a time of incredible changes, both physically and emotionally. As your baby bump grows, so does your excitement about dressing for this special time in your life.

Finding stylish and comfortable maternity clothes can boost your confidence and help you feel your best. Let's explore some tips for navigating maternity fashion with comfort and style.

Embrace Your Changing Body

Your body is doing amazing things, so celebrate it! Embrace your new curves and focus on highlighting your beautiful baby bump. Here's how:

Maternity Basics: Invest in maternity essentials like stretchy leggings, maternity jeans with belly bands, and comfortable maternity bras that provide support without digging into your skin.

Flowy Tops and Tunics: Flowy tops and empire-waist tunics are flattering and comfortable. They drape nicely over your bump and can be dressed up or down depending on the occasion.

Wrap Dresses: Wrap dresses are a maternity wardrobe staple. They adjust to your changing shape and accentuate your curves in all the right places.

Prioritize Comfort

Comfort is key during pregnancy, especially as your body adjusts to its new shape. Here are some tips for staying comfortable without sacrificing style:

Breathable Fabrics: Opt for natural, breathable fabrics like cotton and jersey. They allow your skin to breathe and provide comfort throughout the day.

Stretchy Waistbands: Look for maternity bottoms with stretchy waistbands that can be adjusted as your bump grows. Elastic panels and drawstrings are practical options.

Flat Shoes: As your pregnancy progresses, your center of gravity shifts. Choose supportive, flat shoes or low-heeled options to reduce strain on your back and feet.

Layer Up

Pregnancy hormones can cause fluctuations in body temperature. Layering allows you to adjust your clothing to stay comfortable:

Lightweight Cardigans: Cardigans are versatile and can be layered over tops or dresses. Opt for lightweight fabrics that can be easily removed if you get too warm.

Versatile Scarves: Scarves add style and can be used for warmth or as a nursing cover later on. Choose soft, breathable fabrics that feel comfortable against your skin.

Dress for the Occasion

Whether you're attending a casual brunch or a formal event, there are maternity options for every occasion:

Casual Wear: Keep it simple with maternity tees, leggings, and comfortable flats or sneakers. Add accessories like a statement necklace or earrings to elevate your look.

Workwear: If you're still working during pregnancy, invest in maternity trousers, skirts, or dresses that provide professional comfort. Pair with blouses or shirts that allow room for your growing belly.

Special Occasions: Don't be afraid to dress up for special events! Maternity maxi dresses or evening gowns with empire waists are elegant options that ensure you look and feel amazing.

Personalize Your Style

Above all, maternity fashion is about expressing your unique style and feeling confident. Experiment with colors, patterns, and accessories that reflect your personality:

Accessories: Add pops of color with scarves, belts, or statement jewelry. Accessories can instantly elevate a simple outfit and make it feel more polished.

Hair and Makeup: Pamper yourself with a new hairstyle or experiment with makeup techniques that enhance your pregnancy glow.

Comfortable Undergarments: Invest in supportive maternity bras and underwear that fit well and provide the support you need. Your body is changing, so prioritize comfort and fit.

Shop Smart

Maternity clothes don't have to break the bank. Here are some tips for shopping smart:

Shop Sales and Clearance: Look for maternity wear on sale or in clearance sections. Online retailers often offer discounts, especially during seasonal sales.

Borrow or Swap: Consider borrowing maternity clothes from friends or family members who have recently been pregnant. You can also participate in clothing swaps with other expecting mums.

Invest in Versatile Pieces: Choose maternity clothes that can be mixed and matched to create multiple outfits. Versatility allows you to maximize your wardrobe without buying too many pieces.

Celebrate Your Pregnancy Journey

Maternity fashion is an opportunity to celebrate this special time in your life. Embrace the changes, pamper yourself with comfortable and stylish clothing, and enjoy expressing your personal style.

Remember, the most important thing is to feel confident and comfortable in whatever you wear.

Your Third Trimester (Weeks 27-40)

The Home Stretch: Preparing for Birth

You're in the home stretch, mama! The third trimester is an exciting and sometimes nerve-wracking time as you prepare to meet your little one.

There's so much to think about, but don't worry – we've got you covered with some helpful tips to make sure you're ready for the big day.

Creating Your Birth Plan

A birth plan is a great way to communicate your preferences for labor and delivery with your healthcare team.

It's not set in stone, but it helps guide your caregivers in understanding your wishes. Here's what to consider:

Labor Preferences: Think about where you want to give birth (hospital, birthing center, home) and who you want to be there with you. Consider your preferences for pain management, such as epidurals, natural pain relief methods, or medication-free options.

Delivery Preferences: Consider whether you want a vaginal birth or are open to a cesarean if necessary. Think about positions for labor and delivery, as well as any tools or methods you'd like to use, such as birthing balls, water births, or specific breathing techniques.

Postpartum Care: Outline your preferences for immediate postpartum care, including delayed cord clamping, skin-to-skin contact, and breastfeeding initiation.

Flexibility: Remember, birth plans should be flexible. Situations can change, and it's important to be open to adjustments for the safety of both you and your baby.

Packing Your Hospital Bag

Having a well-packed hospital bag can make your stay more comfortable. Here's a checklist to get you started:

For You: Comfortable clothing, a robe, nursing bras, socks, slippers, toiletries, hair ties, lip balm, and any personal comfort items like a pillow or blanket.

For Baby: Onesies, a going-home outfit, a hat, socks, mittens, swaddles, and a blanket. Don't forget the car seat!

For Your Partner: Comfortable clothing, toiletries, snacks, a camera or phone for pictures, and any necessary chargers.

Important Documents: Your ID, insurance information, and any hospital paperwork.

Preparing Your Home

Getting your home ready for your baby's arrival can help reduce stress and make the transition smoother:

Nesting: Many expectant mums experience a burst of energy and the urge to prepare their home. Use this time to organize the nursery, wash baby clothes, and stock up on diapers and wipes.

Safety First: Ensure your home is baby-proofed. Secure furniture, cover outlets, and remove any hazards from areas where your baby will spend time.

Meal Prep: Consider preparing and freezing meals ahead of time. This will make it easier to have nutritious meals on hand during those busy first weeks with your newborn.

Cleaning: A clean home can make for a more relaxing environment. Consider hiring a cleaning service or enlisting friends and family to help with deep cleaning before baby arrives.

Taking Care of Yourself

Your well-being is crucial as you approach the final weeks of pregnancy:

Rest: Get as much rest as you can. Listen to your body and take naps when needed. Pillows can help support your belly and back for a more comfortable sleep.

Hydration and Nutrition: Continue to eat a balanced diet and drink plenty of water. Small, frequent meals can help if you're experiencing heartburn or discomfort.

Exercise: Gentle exercise, like walking or prenatal yoga, can help keep you active and ease some pregnancy discomforts. Always check with your healthcare provider before starting any new exercise routine.

Mental Health: It's normal to feel a mix of excitement and anxiety as your due date approaches.

Practice relaxation techniques such as deep breathing, meditation, or prenatal massage. Talk to your partner, friends, or a counselor if you're feeling overwhelmed.

Educating Yourself

Knowledge is empowering. Spend some time learning about labor, delivery, and newborn care:

Prenatal Classes: Consider taking a prenatal class with your partner. Topics often include stages of labor, pain management, breastfeeding, and newborn care.

Books and Resources: Read books or online resources about childbirth and infant care. Knowledge can help reduce anxiety and prepare you for what to expect.

Creating Your Birth Plan

As your due date approaches, you might be thinking more about what you want your labor and delivery experience to be like.

Creating a birth plan is a great way to communicate your preferences and desires to your healthcare team, ensuring that your birthing experience is as close to your vision as possible.

Think of it as a roadmap for one of the most important journeys of your life. Let's walk through the steps to creating a thoughtful and flexible birth plan.

Understanding What a Birth Plan Is

A birth plan is a document that outlines your preferences for labor, delivery, and postpartum care. It's a way to communicate your wishes to your healthcare providers and support team.

While it's important to have a plan, it's equally important to stay flexible, as labor can be unpredictable, and the safety of you and your baby comes first.

Start with the Basics

Begin your birth plan with basic information:

Your Name and Contact Information: Include your name, due date, and contact information.

Healthcare Provider: List your doctor or midwife's name and contact information.

Birth Location: Specify where you plan to give birth (hospital, birthing center, home).

Support Persons: Include the names of your partner, doula, or any other support persons who will be with you during labor.

Preferences for Labor

Outline your preferences for how you'd like labor to progress:

Environment: Describe the atmosphere you prefer (dim lighting, music, aromatherapy).

Mobility: Indicate whether you'd like the freedom to move around during labor.

Positions: Specify any labor positions you prefer, such as walking, sitting, or using a birthing ball.

Hydration and Nutrition: Note if you'd like to drink fluids or eat light snacks during labor, if permitted by your provider.

Monitoring: State your preference for continuous or intermittent fetal monitoring.

Pain Management

Detail your preferences for managing pain during labor:

Natural Pain Relief: List any non-medical pain relief methods you'd like to use, such as breathing techniques, hydrotherapy, or massage.

Medical Pain Relief: Specify whether you're open to medications such as epidurals, nitrous oxide, or other analgesics. If you have strong feelings either way, make sure to include them.

Delivery Preferences

Describe your preferences for the actual delivery:

Positions for Pushing: Indicate if you have a preferred position for pushing (squatting, side-lying, on hands and knees).

Assisted Delivery: State your thoughts on assisted delivery methods, such as the use of forceps or vacuum extraction.

Episiotomy: Note whether you prefer to avoid an episiotomy if possible.

Immediate Postpartum Care

Outline your wishes for the moments following your baby's birth:

Skin-to-Skin Contact: Specify if you'd like immediate skin-to-skin contact with your baby.

Cord Clamping: Indicate whether you'd like delayed cord clamping.

Newborn Procedures: List your preferences for newborn procedures, such as the administration of vitamin K, eye ointment, and first bath.

Breastfeeding: State your intention to breastfeed and any support you might need.

Special Considerations

Include any other special considerations that are important to you:

Cesarean Section: If a cesarean becomes necessary, outline any preferences you have for that experience (e.g., having your partner present, playing music, immediate skin-to-skin).

Cultural or Religious Practices: Note any specific cultural or religious practices you'd like respected during labor and delivery.

Communicate and Review

Once you've drafted your birth plan:

Discuss with Your Provider: Review your birth plan with your healthcare provider. They can provide insights and help ensure your preferences are realistic and safe.

Share with Your Support Team: Make sure your partner, doula, and anyone else involved in your birth experience are familiar with your plan.

Stay Flexible: Remember, a birth plan is a guide, not a guarantee. Be open to changes as circumstances evolve during labor and delivery.

Exercise and Pregnancy: Staying Active Safely

Staying active during pregnancy is one of the best things you can do for yourself and your baby. Exercise helps you maintain a healthy weight, boosts your mood, improves sleep, and can even make labor and delivery easier.

But with all the changes happening in your body, it's important to exercise safely. Let's explore how you can stay active and healthy throughout your pregnancy.

Benefits of Exercise During Pregnancy

First, let's talk about why staying active is so beneficial during pregnancy:

Boosts Energy: Regular exercise can help combat fatigue and give you more energy throughout the day.

Improves Mood: Physical activity releases endorphins, which can help reduce stress and improve your mood.

Promotes Better Sleep: Exercise can help you fall asleep faster and enjoy deeper sleep.

Reduces Discomfort: Staying active can help alleviate common pregnancy discomforts like back pain and constipation.

Prepares for Labor: Strengthening your muscles and improving your cardiovascular health can make labor and delivery easier.

Safe Exercises for Each Trimester

Your exercise routine may need to adapt as your pregnancy progresses. Here are some safe and effective exercises for each trimester:

First Trimester:

Walking: A gentle way to keep active without putting too much strain on your body.

Swimming: Provides a full-body workout and helps alleviate swelling.

Prenatal Yoga: Helps improve flexibility, reduce stress, and promote relaxation.

Strength Training: Light weights or resistance bands can help maintain muscle tone. Focus on proper form and avoid heavy lifting.

Second Trimester:

Walking and Swimming: Continue these low-impact activities.

Prenatal Yoga and Pilates: These exercises help with balance and core strength.

Stationary Cycling: A safe way to get your heart rate up without the risk of falling.

Third Trimester:

Walking and Swimming: Still great options for maintaining activity.

Prenatal Yoga: Focus on relaxation and gentle stretching.

Light Strength Training: Continue with light weights and resistance bands, focusing on maintaining strength without overexerting.

Tips for Safe Exercise During Pregnancy

Here are some essential tips to keep in mind to ensure you're exercising safely:

Consult Your Healthcare Provider: Before starting any exercise program, check with your doctor or midwife to ensure it's safe for you and your baby.

Stay Hydrated: Drink plenty of water before, during, and after exercise to stay hydrated.

Warm Up and Cool Down: Always start with a gentle warm-up and end with a cool-down to prevent injury and help your body transition.

Listen to Your Body: Pay attention to how you feel. If you experience any pain, dizziness, shortness of breath, or any other concerning symptoms, stop exercising and contact your healthcare provider.

Avoid High-Risk Activities: Steer clear of activities with a high risk of falling or abdominal trauma, such as skiing, horseback riding, or contact sports.

Modify as Needed: As your belly grows, you may need to modify your exercises. Avoid exercises that involve lying flat on your back after the first trimester, as this can reduce blood flow to your baby.

Pelvic Floor Exercises

Strengthening your pelvic floor muscles is especially important during pregnancy and postpartum. These muscles support your bladder, uterus, and bowels. Here's how to do pelvic floor exercises (also known as Kegels):

Find the Right Muscles: To identify your pelvic floor muscles, try stopping your urine flow midstream. These are the muscles you want to target.

Practice Regularly: Aim to do pelvic floor exercises several times a day. Tighten the muscles, hold for a few seconds, and then relax. Repeat 10-15 times per session.

Incorporate into Daily Routine: You can do these exercises anywhere – while sitting, standing, or lying down.

Staying Motivated

Staying motivated to exercise during pregnancy can sometimes be challenging, especially if you're dealing with fatigue or morning sickness. Here are some tips to help you stay on track:

Set Realistic Goals: Set small, achievable goals and celebrate your progress.

Find a Buddy: Exercising with a friend or joining a prenatal exercise class can provide support and motivation.

Mix It Up: Keep your routine interesting by trying different types of exercise.

Listen to Your Body: Adjust your routine as needed based on how you're feeling each day.

When to Stop Exercising and Seek Medical Advice

While exercise is generally safe and beneficial during pregnancy, there are certain signs that you should stop exercising and contact your healthcare provider:

Vaginal Bleeding or Fluid Leakage: These could be signs of a complication and should be evaluated immediately.

Dizziness or Fainting: If you feel dizzy or faint, stop exercising and sit down until you feel better.

Chest Pain or Shortness of Breath: These symptoms require immediate medical attention.

Painful Contractions: If you experience regular, painful contractions before 37 weeks, contact your healthcare provider.

Enjoy the Journey

Exercise during pregnancy is about staying healthy and preparing your body for the incredible task of giving birth.

It's not about pushing your limits or achieving fitness goals. Be kind to yourself, listen to your body, and find activities that you enjoy.

This is a special time in your life, and staying active can help you feel your best as you prepare to welcome your little one.

Mental Health: Managing Anxiety and Mood Swings

Pregnancy is an incredible journey filled with excitement, anticipation, and profound changes. But it's also a time when you might experience heightened emotions, anxiety, and mood swings.

These feelings are completely normal and part of the process of becoming a mum.

Let's talk about why this happens and explore some strategies to help you manage your mental health during this transformative time.

Understanding Pregnancy Emotions

First, let's understand why you might be feeling this way:

Hormonal Changes: Pregnancy brings significant hormonal shifts, which can impact your mood and emotions. Higher levels of hormones like estrogen and progesterone can contribute to feelings of anxiety, irritability, and emotional ups and downs.

Physical Changes: Your body is going through rapid changes, which can be overwhelming and sometimes uncomfortable. These changes can affect how you feel mentally and emotionally.

Life Changes: Pregnancy marks a major life transition. Whether it's your first baby or you're adding to your family, the anticipation of becoming a parent can bring a mix of joy and anxiety.

Managing Anxiety

Feeling anxious during pregnancy is common, but there are ways to manage these feelings:

Talk About It: Don't keep your worries to yourself. Talk to your partner, a trusted friend, or a family member about how you're feeling. Sometimes just sharing your thoughts can provide relief.

Seek Professional Help: If your anxiety feels overwhelming, consider talking to a therapist or counselor who specializes in prenatal mental health. They can provide strategies and support tailored to your needs.

Practice Mindfulness: Mindfulness techniques, such as deep breathing, meditation, and yoga, can help you stay grounded and reduce anxiety. Even a few minutes a day can make a big difference.

Stay Informed: Educate yourself about pregnancy and childbirth. Knowing what to expect can help alleviate some of the fears and uncertainties.

Create a Routine: Establishing a daily routine can provide a sense of normalcy and control. Include activities that you enjoy and that help you relax.

Coping with Mood Swings

Mood swings are a natural part of pregnancy, but they can be challenging to deal with. Here are some tips to help manage these emotional fluctuations:

Stay Active: Regular exercise, such as walking, swimming, or prenatal yoga, can boost your mood and reduce stress. Physical activity releases endorphins, which are natural mood lifters.

Get Enough Sleep: Lack of sleep can exacerbate mood swings. Prioritize restful sleep by establishing a bedtime routine and creating a comfortable sleeping environment.

Eat Well: A balanced diet can impact your mood. Eat regular, nutritious meals and stay hydrated. Avoid excessive caffeine and sugary snacks, which can lead to energy crashes.

Stay Connected: Maintain social connections with friends and family. Supportive relationships can provide comfort and stability.

Set Realistic Expectations: Be kind to yourself. It's okay to have days when you feel less than perfect. Set realistic expectations and give yourself permission to rest when needed.

Seeking Support

You don't have to go through this alone. There are many resources available to support your mental health during pregnancy:

Prenatal Classes: Join a prenatal class to connect with other expectant mums and learn more about pregnancy, childbirth, and parenting.

Support Groups: Consider joining a support group for pregnant women. Sharing your experiences with others who understand can be very comforting.

Talk to Your Healthcare Provider: If you're struggling with anxiety or mood swings, talk to your doctor or midwife. They can provide resources and refer you to a mental health professional if needed.

When to Seek Help

It's important to recognize when you might need professional help:

Persistent Anxiety or Depression: If you're feeling anxious or depressed most of the time and it's interfering with your daily life, seek professional help.

Difficulty Functioning: If you're finding it hard to perform daily activities or take care of yourself, reach out for support.

Thoughts of Self-Harm: If you're experiencing thoughts of self-harm or harming your baby, seek immediate help from a healthcare provider or mental health professional.

Signs of Labor: When to Go to the Hospital

As you approach your due date, you might be eagerly anticipating (or maybe a little anxious about) the start of labor.

Knowing the signs of labor and when to head to the hospital can help you feel more prepared and confident as the big day approaches.

 Let's explore the common signs of labor and give you a clear understanding of when it's time to grab your hospital bag and go.

Early Signs of Labor

Your body will give you some clues that labor is approaching, but these signs can sometimes be subtle and gradual:

Lightening: Also known as "dropping," this is when your baby moves lower into your pelvis. You might notice that you can breathe more easily, but you may also feel increased pressure on your bladder.

Increased Discharge: You might notice an increase in vaginal discharge, which can be clear, pink, or slightly bloody. This is often the result of your cervix beginning to efface (thin out) and dilate (open).

Bloody Show: A pink or blood-tinged mucus discharge may indicate that labor is near. This is your mucus plug, which has been protecting your cervix during pregnancy.

Nesting Instinct: A sudden burst of energy and the urge to clean and prepare your home for the baby can be a sign that labor is on the horizon.

True Labor vs. False Labor

It's important to distinguish between true labor and false labor (also known as Braxton Hicks contractions):

Braxton Hicks Contractions: These "practice" contractions can start weeks or even months before your due date. They are usually irregular, don't get closer together, and often go away with rest or hydration.

True Labor Contractions: These contractions are regular, get closer together, increase in intensity, and don't go away with rest. They typically start in the back and move to the front of your abdomen.

Key Signs of Labor

Here are the key signs that indicate you're in labor and it's time to go to the hospital:

Regular Contractions: When you have regular contractions that are about 5 minutes apart and last for about 60 seconds each, it's time to call your healthcare provider and head to the hospital. Use the 5-1-1 rule as a guide: contractions are 5 minutes apart, lasting 1 minute each, for at least 1 hour.

Water Breaking: If your amniotic sac ruptures and you experience a gush or a steady trickle of fluid, it's time to go to the hospital, even if you're not having contractions yet. Note the color and odor of the fluid and inform your healthcare provider.

Intense Pain or Pressure: If you experience intense pain or pressure in your pelvis or back, or if you're unable to walk or talk through contractions, it's a sign that labor is progressing, and you should go to the hospital.

Bleeding: If you experience heavy vaginal bleeding, go to the hospital immediately. Light spotting or a pink discharge can be normal, but heavy bleeding is not and needs immediate medical attention.

Reduced Fetal Movement: If you notice a significant decrease in your baby's movements, contact your healthcare provider right away. Your baby should remain active throughout labor.

When to Call Your Healthcare Provider

In addition to the signs above, call your healthcare provider if you experience:

Severe Headache: A severe headache that doesn't go away with rest or medication.

Blurred Vision or Dizziness: These can be signs of preeclampsia, a serious condition that requires immediate attention.

Sudden Swelling: Rapid or sudden swelling of your face, hands, or feet.

High Fever: A fever of 100.4°F (38°C) or higher.

Preparing for the Hospital

As you approach your due date, it's helpful to have your hospital bag packed and ready to go. Here's a quick checklist of items to include:

Important Documents: ID, insurance information, and your birth plan.

Comfort Items: Your own pillow, a cozy blanket, and items that help you relax (e.g., music, essential oils).

Clothing: Comfortable clothing for labor, a robe, slippers, and a going-home outfit for you and the baby.

Toiletries: Toothbrush, toothpaste, hairbrush, lip balm, and other personal hygiene items.

Snacks and Drinks: Light snacks and drinks for you and your support person.

Baby Essentials: A going-home outfit, blanket, and car seat.

Trust Your Instincts

Every pregnancy and labor experience is unique. Trust your instincts and listen to your body. If something doesn't feel right or you're unsure about what you're experiencing, don't hesitate to call your healthcare provider or go to the hospital. It's always better to be safe and get checked out.

Knowing the signs of labor and when to go to the hospital can help you feel more prepared and less anxious as you approach your due date. Keep your healthcare provider's contact information handy, and don't be afraid to reach out with any questions or concerns.

Understanding Different Birth Scenarios

Every birth is unique, and while you may have a clear vision of how you want your labor and delivery to go, it's essential to be prepared for different scenarios.

Understanding the various ways your baby might enter the world can help you feel more confident and ready for whatever comes your way. Let's explore some common birth scenarios and what to expect with each.

Vaginal Birth

A vaginal birth is the most common type of delivery and what many expectant mums plan for. Here's what to expect:

Stages of Labor: Labor is typically divided into three stages. The first stage involves early labor, active labor, and transition. The second stage is the pushing phase, and the third stage is the delivery of the placenta.

Pain Relief Options: You can choose from various pain relief methods, including natural techniques (breathing exercises, movement, water therapy), medication (like an epidural), or a combination of both.

Delivery: During the second stage, you'll push with each contraction to help your baby move through the birth canal. Your healthcare provider will guide and support you through this process.

Cesarean Section (C-Section)

A C-section is a surgical procedure used to deliver a baby through incisions made in the abdomen and uterus. It might be planned ahead of time or become necessary during labor. Here's what to expect:

Planned C-Section: This is scheduled in advance, often due to medical reasons such as a breech baby, placenta previa, or previous C-sections.

Unplanned C-Section: Sometimes, a C-section becomes necessary during labor due to complications like fetal distress or stalled labor.

Procedure: You'll receive anesthesia (usually a spinal block or epidural) to numb the lower half of your body. Your doctor will make incisions and deliver your baby.

The procedure typically takes about 45 minutes to an hour.

Recovery: Recovery from a C-section generally takes longer than from a vaginal birth. You'll need to take it easy for a few weeks and avoid heavy lifting.

Induced Labor

Induction is the process of stimulating labor artificially. Your healthcare provider might recommend induction for various reasons, such as being overdue, having certain medical conditions, or if there are concerns about your baby's health.

Here's what to expect:

Methods of Induction: Induction methods can include medication (like Pitocin), breaking your water (amniotomy), or using a Foley catheter to help dilate your cervix.

Labor Process: Induced labor can sometimes be more intense than natural labor, but it follows the same stages. Your healthcare provider will closely monitor you and your baby throughout the process.

Vaginal Birth After Cesarean (VBAC)

If you've had a previous C-section, you might be a candidate for a VBAC, which is a vaginal birth after cesarean. Here's what to expect:

Eligibility: Not all women are candidates for VBAC. Factors like the type of incision from your previous C-section, the reason for your previous C-section, and your overall health will be considered.

Risks and Benefits: VBAC carries both risks and benefits. It's important to discuss these with your healthcare provider to make an informed decision.

Labor Process: If you attempt a VBAC, your labor will be closely monitored. In the event of complications, a repeat C-section may become necessary.

Assisted Vaginal Birth

Sometimes, assistance is needed during a vaginal birth to help your baby be born safely. This can include the use of forceps or a vacuum extractor. Here's what to expect:

Forceps: These are tong-like instruments used to gently guide your baby's head out of the birth canal.

Vacuum Extraction: A suction cup is applied to your baby's head to help guide them out during a contraction.

Why It's Needed: Assisted delivery may be necessary if labor isn't progressing, if there are concerns about your baby's heart rate, or if you're too exhausted to push effectively.

Recovery: You may experience some additional soreness and swelling with an assisted birth, but these usually resolve with time.

Water Birth

A water birth involves giving birth in a tub of warm water. Some women choose this option because it can provide pain relief and a more relaxing environment. Here's what to expect:

Environment: Water births can take place at home, in a birthing center, or in some hospitals.

Benefits: Warm water can help you relax, reduce pain, and provide a sense of buoyancy.

Considerations: Not all women are candidates for water birth, especially if there are complications. Discuss this option with your healthcare provider.

Home Birth

Some women choose to give birth at home, attended by a midwife or other qualified healthcare professional. Here's what to expect:

Preparation: You'll need to plan ahead, including setting up a birthing space and having necessary supplies on hand.

Support Team: A skilled midwife and possibly a doula will support you through labor and delivery.

Considerations: Home birth is typically recommended for low-risk pregnancies. It's essential to have a backup plan in case a transfer to a hospital becomes necessary.

Embrace Flexibility

While it's great to have a birth plan and preferences, it's also important to stay flexible. Labor and delivery can be unpredictable, and the primary goal is a safe and healthy delivery for both you and your baby.

Understanding the different birth scenarios can help you feel more prepared and confident as you approach your due date. Each birth is unique, and what matters most is that you and your baby are safe and healthy. Trust your healthcare team, listen to your body, and remember that every step you take brings you closer to meeting your precious little one.

Meeting Your Baby: First Moments and Bonding

The moment you've been dreaming about is finally here – meeting your baby for the first time. This is a truly magical and emotional experience, filled with wonder and love.

The First Cry

The sound of your baby's first cry is one you'll never forget. It signals the beginning of their life outside the womb and reassures you that they're breathing well.

Don't worry if your baby doesn't cry immediately; some babies are quieter than others. The healthcare team will ensure your baby is healthy and breathing properly.

Skin-to-Skin Contact

One of the best ways to start bonding with your baby is through skin-to-skin contact. Here's why it's so special:

Benefits: Skin-to-skin contact helps regulate your baby's body temperature, heart rate, and breathing. It also promotes breastfeeding and provides comfort and security for your newborn.

How to Do It: Simply place your baby, dressed in just a diaper, on your bare chest. Cover both of you with a blanket to keep warm. Enjoy these intimate moments, and let your baby feel your heartbeat and warmth.

The Golden Hour

The first hour after birth, often called the "Golden Hour," is a critical time for bonding and establishing breastfeeding. Here's what you can expect:

Quiet Time: Hospitals and birthing centers often try to minimize interruptions during this time to allow you and your baby to bond.

First Breastfeeding: If you plan to breastfeed, this is an excellent time to start. Your baby may show interest in nursing, and the early colostrum is packed with nutrients and antibodies.

Eye Contact and Communication

Your baby's vision is still developing, but they can see your face when held close. Making eye contact and talking to your baby helps strengthen your bond:

Eye Contact: Hold your baby close and look into their eyes. They'll be drawn to your face and voice.

Talking and Singing: Your voice is familiar and soothing to your baby. Talk to them, sing lullabies, and enjoy these first conversations.

Emotional Roller Coaster

Meeting your baby can be an emotional whirlwind. You might feel overwhelming love, relief, exhaustion, and even a bit of anxiety. All these emotions are normal:

Love and Joy: The overwhelming love and joy you feel when you first hold your baby is indescribable.

Tears: It's completely normal to shed tears of joy or relief. Allow yourself to feel and express your emotions.

Anxiety: It's natural to feel a bit anxious about your new role as a parent. Remember, you're not alone, and it's okay to ask for help.

Bonding for Partners

Bonding isn't just for mums; partners can also create a strong connection with the baby:

Skin-to-Skin Contact: Partners can also do skin-to-skin contact to bond with the baby.

Holding and Talking: Spend time holding your baby and talking to them. Your voice and touch are incredibly comforting.

Supporting Mum: Supporting the new mum during this time strengthens your bond as a family and helps create a loving environment for your baby.

Recognizing Your Baby's Needs

Newborns have their own ways of communicating. Learning to recognize and respond to your baby's cues helps build trust and strengthens your bond:

Crying: Babies cry to communicate their needs. Over time, you'll start to recognize different types of cries for hunger, discomfort, or sleepiness.

Feeding Cues: Look for signs that your baby is hungry, such as rooting (turning their head towards you with an open mouth), sucking on their hands, or making smacking noises.

Comfort Needs: Sometimes, your baby just needs to be held and comforted. Holding, rocking, and gentle shushing can help soothe them.

Taking Care of Yourself

Your well-being is crucial during this time. Taking care of yourself enables you to care for your baby:

Rest: Try to rest whenever you can, even if it's just short naps. Sleep deprivation is common, but rest helps you recharge.

Nutrition: Eating well helps you recover from childbirth and maintain your energy levels, especially if you're breastfeeding.

Support: Don't hesitate to ask for help from your partner, family, or friends. It's okay to take breaks and take care of your own needs.

Meeting your baby for the first time is a moment filled with pure magic and joy. These initial moments of bonding lay the foundation for a loving and secure relationship. Embrace the emotions, take it one step at a time, and remember that it's a learning process for both you and your baby.

You're embarking on an incredible journey of parenthood. Trust yourself, lean on your support system, and cherish these beautiful first moments with your precious little one.

Your Postpartum Body: Healing and Recovery

Congratulations, mama! You've brought your beautiful baby into the world. While you're likely focused on caring for your little one, it's equally important to take care of yourself.

Your body has gone through an incredible journey, and now it's time to focus on healing and recovery. Let's talk about what you can expect from your postpartum body and how to support your recovery.

Immediate Postpartum Changes

Right after birth, your body begins the process of healing and adjusting. Here's what you can expect in the immediate postpartum period:

Afterpains: You might experience cramping as your uterus contracts back to its pre-pregnancy size. These afterpains are more noticeable if you're breastfeeding, as nursing triggers the release of oxytocin, which helps your uterus contract.

Bleeding (Lochia): You'll have vaginal bleeding and discharge, called lochia, which is your body's way of shedding the lining of your uterus. It starts off heavy and bright red, gradually becoming lighter and more pinkish-brown over a few weeks.

Perineal Soreness: If you had a vaginal birth, your perineum (the area between your vagina and anus) might be sore, especially if you had any tears or an episiotomy. Ice packs, witch hazel pads, and sitz baths can help soothe the discomfort.

C-Section Recovery

If you had a cesarean section, your recovery will involve caring for your incision and managing post-surgery discomfort:

Incision Care: Keep your incision clean and dry. Follow your healthcare provider's instructions for caring for your stitches or staples.

Pain Management: You'll likely experience soreness around the incision site. Take prescribed pain medications as directed and avoid heavy lifting or strenuous activities.

Movement: Gentle movement is important to prevent blood clots. Take short walks around your home as you feel able, and gradually increase your activity level.

Breastfeeding and Breast Care

Breastfeeding can bring its own set of challenges and changes:

Milk Production: Your milk will come in a few days after birth, leading to fullness or engorgement. Frequent nursing or pumping can help relieve discomfort.

Nipple Soreness: It's common to experience some nipple soreness, especially in the early days. Use lanolin cream, and ensure your baby is latching correctly.

Breast Infections: Watch for signs of mastitis (breast infection), such as redness, swelling, and flu-like symptoms. If you suspect an infection, contact your healthcare provider.

Physical Changes and Self-Care

Your body will continue to change in the weeks and months after birth. Here are some key aspects of postpartum self-care:

Rest and Sleep: Rest is crucial for your recovery. Nap when your baby naps, and don't hesitate to ask for help from your partner, family, or friends.

Hydration and Nutrition: Drink plenty of water and eat a balanced diet rich in fruits, vegetables, whole grains, and lean proteins. Proper nutrition supports healing and energy levels.

Pelvic Floor Exercises: Gentle pelvic floor exercises (Kegels) can help strengthen your pelvic muscles and support recovery from vaginal birth.

Gentle Exercise: Start with light activities like walking when you feel ready. Avoid strenuous exercise until your healthcare provider gives you the go-ahead.

Emotional Well-Being

Your emotional health is just as important as your physical recovery:

Baby Blues: It's normal to experience mood swings, sadness, or anxiety in the first couple of weeks after birth, often referred to as the "baby blues." These feelings are usually temporary and related to hormonal changes and the adjustment to motherhood.

Postpartum Depression: If you're experiencing persistent feelings of sadness, hopelessness, or anxiety that interfere with your daily life, you might be dealing with postpartum depression. It's important to seek help from your healthcare provider or a mental health professional.

Self-Compassion: Be kind to yourself. Recovery takes time, and it's okay to have mixed emotions.

Give yourself grace and don't pressure yourself to "bounce back" quickly.

When to Seek Help

Contact your healthcare provider if you experience any of the following:

Heavy Bleeding: Soaking through a pad in an hour or passing large clots.

Signs of Infection: Fever, chills, severe pain, or foul-smelling discharge.

Severe Pain: Persistent or worsening pain that isn't relieved by medication.

Mental Health Concerns: Persistent feelings of sadness, anxiety, or hopelessness.

Your postpartum recovery is a unique journey, just like your pregnancy and birth. It's a time for healing, bonding with your baby, and adjusting to your new role as a mother.

Listen to your body, prioritize self-care, and lean on your support network.

You're doing an amazing job, mama. Take it one day at a time, celebrate the small victories, and remember that healing is a gradual process.

You've brought new life into the world, and now it's time to take care of yourself with the same love and care you're giving to your baby.

Breastfeeding Basics: Tips and Troubleshooting

Breastfeeding can be a beautiful and rewarding way to nourish and bond with your baby, but it can also come with its challenges.

Whether you're a first-time mum or looking for a refresher, this chapter will provide you with the basics of breastfeeding, tips for success, and troubleshooting common issues. Let's dive in!

The First Feed

The first breastfeeding session often happens within the first hour after birth, during what's known as the "Golden Hour." Here's how to get started:

Skin-to-Skin Contact: Holding your baby skin-to-skin helps regulate their body temperature, promotes bonding, and encourages the natural breastfeeding instinct.

Latch: To help your baby latch, hold them close, and gently guide their mouth to your nipple. A good latch is crucial for effective feeding and comfort.

Colostrum: Your first milk, called colostrum, is rich in nutrients and antibodies. It's often called "liquid gold" for its many benefits to your baby's health.

Finding the Right Position

Finding a comfortable breastfeeding position is key. Here are a few popular ones:

Cradle Hold: Hold your baby in your arm, with their head resting in the crook of your elbow and their body facing yours. Support your breast with your opposite hand.

Football Hold: Hold your baby at your side, tucking them under your arm like a football, with their legs pointing towards your back. This position can be helpful for mums who had a C-section.

Side-Lying Position: Lie on your side with your baby facing you. This position can be restful for nighttime feedings.

Laid-Back Position: Recline comfortably, and place your baby on your chest. Let them find their way to your breast and latch on naturally.

Recognizing Hunger Cues

Babies give signals when they're ready to feed. Look for these early hunger cues to know when it's time:

Rooting: Turning their head towards your hand or breast with an open mouth.

Sucking on Hands: Bringing hands to their mouth and sucking.

Fussiness: Increased movement and mild fussing.

Crying: Crying is a late hunger cue; it's best to start feeding before your baby reaches this stage.

Ensuring a Good Latch

A good latch is essential for effective breastfeeding and preventing discomfort. Here's how to achieve it:

Align Your Baby: Make sure your baby's nose is opposite your nipple. This helps them open their mouth wide and take in a good amount of the areola.

Tickle the Lip: Use your nipple to tickle your baby's upper lip, encouraging them to open wide.

Bring Baby to Breast: When their mouth is wide open, bring your baby to your breast (not the other way around). Ensure their chin touches your breast first.

Feeding Frequency and Duration

Newborns typically need to feed every 2-3 hours, including during the night. Here's what to expect:

On-Demand Feeding: Respond to your baby's hunger cues rather than sticking to a strict schedule. This helps establish a good milk supply.

Duration: Let your baby nurse until they release the breast or fall asleep. This can be anywhere from 10 to 45 minutes per feeding.

Cluster Feeding: Your baby might have periods of frequent feeding, known as cluster feeding, often in the evening. This is normal and helps increase your milk supply.

Common Breastfeeding Challenges

Breastfeeding can come with challenges, but knowing how to address them can help you overcome them:

Sore Nipples: Ensure a proper latch, and use lanolin cream or breast milk to soothe soreness. If pain persists, consult a lactation consultant.

Engorgement: If your breasts are overly full and uncomfortable, try feeding more frequently, using warm compresses before feeding, and expressing a small amount of milk to soften the breast.

Blocked Ducts: Apply warm compresses, massage the area gently, and ensure your baby is nursing effectively to clear the blockage.

Mastitis: If you develop flu-like symptoms, redness, and pain in your breast, you might have mastitis, a breast infection. Continue breastfeeding and contact your healthcare provider for treatment.

Tips for Successful Breastfeeding

Here are some additional tips to support your breastfeeding journey:

Stay Hydrated: Drink plenty of water to stay hydrated and support milk production.

Eat Well: A balanced diet with plenty of nutrients helps you produce quality milk and maintain your energy levels.

Rest: Rest whenever you can. Sleep deprivation is common, but try to nap when your baby naps.

Seek Support: Join a breastfeeding support group or connect with a lactation consultant if you need help or encouragement.

When to Seek Help

Don't hesitate to seek help if you encounter any issues or have concerns about breastfeeding:

Painful Latch: If you experience ongoing pain during breastfeeding, consult a lactation consultant.

Low Milk Supply: If you're worried about your milk supply, your baby's weight gain, or feeding frequency, reach out to your healthcare provider.

Emotional Support: Breastfeeding can be emotionally challenging. Seek support from friends, family, or a support group.

Breastfeeding is a journey that comes with its ups and downs. Be patient with yourself and your baby as you both learn and adjust. Remember that it's okay to ask for help and that every bit of breast milk you provide is a wonderful gift to your baby.

Navigating the Newborn Stage: Sleep, Feeding, and Soothing

Welcome to the newborn stage, a time filled with incredible joy, sleepless nights, and many precious moments. This period can be both magical and overwhelming as you and your baby get to know each other.

Let's explore some essential tips for navigating sleep, feeding, and soothing your newborn to help make this time a little easier and even more special.

Understanding Newborn Sleep Patterns

Newborns sleep a lot, but not always in predictable patterns. Here's what you need to know about their sleep:

Frequent Sleep Cycles: Newborns typically sleep for 14-17 hours a day, but this is broken into short stretches of 2-4 hours, both day and night.

Light Sleep: They spend a lot of time in REM (rapid eye movement) sleep, which is lighter and more prone to waking. This stage is essential for brain development.

Safe Sleep Practices: Always place your baby on their back to sleep, use a firm mattress, and keep the crib free of soft bedding, pillows, and toys to reduce the risk of SIDS (Sudden Infant Death Syndrome).

Establishing a Sleep Routine

While newborns aren't ready for a strict sleep schedule, you can start establishing a gentle routine to help them feel secure:

Create a Calm Environment: Dim the lights, use a white noise machine, and keep the room at a comfortable temperature.

Consistent Cues: Begin to introduce consistent cues for sleep, such as a warm bath, a gentle massage, or a lullaby before putting your baby down.

Follow Sleepy Cues: Look for signs that your baby is tired, such as yawning, rubbing eyes, or fussiness, and put them to sleep before they become overtired.

Feeding Your Newborn

Feeding is a crucial part of caring for your newborn, whether you're breastfeeding, formula feeding, or a combination of both:

On-Demand Feeding: Newborns need to eat frequently, about every 2-3 hours. Watch for hunger cues like rooting, sucking on hands, or fussiness.

Breastfeeding: Aim for 8-12 feedings in 24 hours. Trust your baby to know how much they need; frequent nursing helps establish your milk supply.

Formula Feeding: Offer 1.5 to 3 ounces of formula every 2-3 hours. Your baby's intake will gradually increase as they grow.

Burping: Burp your baby during and after feedings to help release any swallowed air and reduce fussiness.

Soothing Techniques for a Fussy Baby

Newborns cry as their primary way of communicating. Here are some soothing techniques to help calm your baby:

Swaddling: Wrapping your baby snugly in a blanket can provide comfort and mimic the feeling of the womb.

White Noise: The sound of a white noise machine, a fan, or even a gentle shushing sound can help soothe your baby.

Movement: Rocking, swaying, or gentle bouncing can be very calming. You can also try taking your baby for a walk in a stroller or a car ride.

Sucking: Many babies find sucking to be very soothing. Offer a pacifier or let your baby suck on their fingers or your breast.

The newborn stage is a time of learning, adjustment, and incredible bonding. While it can be challenging, remember that it's also a time of immense growth and love.

Trust your instincts, be patient with yourself and your baby, and take things one day at a time.

Handling Baby Blues and Postpartum Depression

Bringing a new life into the world is a profound and transformative experience. While it's often filled with joy and wonder, it can also bring unexpected emotional challenges.

It's completely normal to have periods of sadness, anxiety, and overwhelm as you adjust to motherhood.

Understanding the Baby Blues

The baby blues are common and affect up to 80% of new mums. Here's what you need to know:

What Are the Baby Blues? The baby blues are characterized by mood swings, weepiness, irritability, and anxiety. These feelings typically start a few days after birth and can last for up to two weeks.

Causes: Hormonal changes, lack of sleep, physical recovery, and the overwhelming responsibility of caring for a newborn can all contribute to the baby blues.

Symptoms: Feeling sad or overwhelmed, crying for no apparent reason, impatience, irritability, restlessness, and trouble sleeping, even when the baby is asleep.

Coping with the Baby Blues

While the baby blues usually resolve on their own, there are ways to manage your feelings and find some relief:

Rest and Sleep: Prioritize rest and sleep whenever you can. Nap when your baby naps and ask for help from your partner, family, or friends to get more sleep.

Light Exercise: Gentle exercise, such as a walk outside, can boost your mood and provide a much-needed change of scenery.

Emotional Support: Talk to your partner, family, or friends about how you're feeling. Sometimes just sharing your thoughts and concerns can make a big difference.

Recognizing Postpartum Depression

Postpartum depression (PPD) is more severe than the baby blues and affects about 10-20% of new mums. It's important to recognize the signs and seek help:

What Is Postpartum Depression? PPD is a type of depression that can occur after childbirth. It's more intense and longer-lasting than the baby blues and can interfere with your ability to care for yourself and your baby.

Symptoms: Persistent sadness, severe mood swings, excessive crying, difficulty bonding with your baby, withdrawal from family and friends, loss of appetite, insomnia or excessive sleeping, overwhelming fatigue, feelings of worthlessness or guilt, and thoughts of harming yourself or your baby.

Risk Factors: A history of depression or anxiety, stressful life events, lack of support, and hormonal changes can all increase the risk of PPD.

Seeking Help for Postpartum Depression

If you think you might have PPD, it's important to seek help. Here's what you can do:

Talk to Your Healthcare Provider: Your doctor or midwife can provide a diagnosis and discuss treatment options with you.

Reach Out for Support: Don't be afraid to ask for help from your partner, family, and friends. Let them know what you're going through and how they can support you.

Counseling and Therapy: Speaking with a mental health professional can help you work through your feelings and develop coping strategies.

Taking Care of Your Mental Health

Self-Compassion: Be gentle with yourself. Adjusting to motherhood is a significant transition, and it's okay to have mixed emotions.

Set Realistic Expectations: Give yourself permission to let go of perfection. Focus on small accomplishments and celebrate them.

Find Time for Yourself: Even a few minutes of "me time" can make a difference. Take a relaxing bath, read a book, or enjoy a hobby you love.

Connect with Others: Maintain social connections, even if it's just a phone call or a chat with a neighbor. Social support is vital for mental health.

Recognizing When to Seek Immediate Help

In some cases, PPD can lead to more serious conditions, such as postpartum psychosis, which requires immediate medical attention:

Postpartum Psychosis: This is a rare but severe condition that can include symptoms such as hallucinations, delusions, extreme agitation, and confusion. If you or someone you know is experiencing these symptoms, seek emergency medical care right away.

Emergency Signs: It is very important that you seek help immediately from a healthcare provider or call emergency services if you find yourself having thoughts of harming yourself or your baby.

Navigating the emotional landscape of new motherhood can be challenging, but you are not alone.

The baby blues are common, and postpartum depression is a treatable condition. By seeking support and taking care of your mental health, you can find a path to feeling better.

Establishing Routines: Finding Your Rhythm

Life with a newborn can feel like a whirlwind of feedings, diaper changes, and sleepless nights. Amidst all the chaos, establishing routines can bring a sense of order and predictability to your days.

The Importance of Routines

Routines can provide a comforting structure for both you and your baby. Here's why they matter:

Security and Predictability: Consistent routines help your baby feel secure and understand what to expect next, reducing fussiness and anxiety.

Better Sleep Patterns: Establishing a bedtime routine can help signal to your baby that it's time to sleep, promoting better sleep habits.

Bonding Time: Routines create opportunities for regular bonding moments, whether through feeding, playtime, or bath time.

Parental Confidence: Having a routine can help you feel more in control and confident in your parenting, making it easier to manage daily tasks and responsibilities.

Starting with Simple Routines

In the early weeks, your routines will be simple and flexible. Here's how to get started:

Feeding Routine: Whether you're breastfeeding or formula feeding, try to establish a regular feeding pattern. Feed your baby on demand, and gradually, you'll notice a natural rhythm developing.

Sleep Routine: Pay attention to your baby's sleep cues and create a soothing bedtime routine. This could include a warm bath, a gentle massage, a lullaby, and dimming the lights.

Diaper Changes: Incorporate diaper changes into your routine, such as after each feeding or nap.

Keep everything you need nearby to make changes quick and easy.

Creating a Bedtime Routine

A consistent bedtime routine can help your baby wind down and prepare for sleep. Here's a simple routine to consider:

Wind-Down Time: Start with a quiet activity to signal the beginning of the bedtime routine. This could be reading a story, singing a lullaby, or cuddling in a dimly lit room.

Bath Time: A warm bath can be relaxing and help your baby understand that bedtime is approaching.

Massage and Pajamas: After the bath, give your baby a gentle massage with baby lotion, then dress them in comfortable pajamas.

Feeding: Offer a final feed to help your baby feel full and content before sleep.

Sleep Environment: Create a calming sleep environment with a darkened room, white noise, and a comfortable crib.

Finding Your Daytime Rhythm

During the day, focus on establishing a flexible routine that works for you and your baby:

Morning Wake-Up: Try to start the day around the same time each morning. Open the curtains to let in natural light and signal the start of the day.

Playtime: Include periods of play and interaction throughout the day. Tummy time, gentle music, and age-appropriate toys can help stimulate your baby's development.

Nap Times: Pay attention to your baby's sleep cues and offer naps when they seem tired. Over time, you'll notice patterns that can help you predict when they'll need to rest.

Adapting as Your Baby Grows

Remember that routines will change as your baby grows and their needs evolve. Here's how to adapt:

Stay Flexible: Be open to adjusting routines as needed. Growth spurts, teething, and developmental milestones can all affect your baby's patterns.

Observe and Adjust: Pay attention to your baby's cues and adjust routines accordingly. If a particular routine isn't working, don't be afraid to change it up.

Introduce New Activities: As your baby gets older, incorporate new activities into your routine, such as storytime, outdoor walks, or baby classes.

Finding What Works for You

Every family is unique, and there's no one-size-fits-all approach to routines. Here's how to find what works best for you:

Trial and Error: Be patient and willing to experiment with different routines. What works one week might need tweaking the next.

Trust Your Instincts: You know your baby best. Trust your instincts and make adjustments based on what feels right for both of you.

Celebrate Small Wins: Celebrate the small victories, whether it's a smooth bedtime or a peaceful feeding session. Each positive experience helps build your confidence.

Establishing routines is a gradual process that requires patience and flexibility. The goal is to create a nurturing environment where both you and your baby feel comfortable and secure.

Returning to Work: Balancing Motherhood and Career

Returning to work after having a baby is a significant transition, filled with a mix of emotions. You might feel excited to reconnect with your professional self, yet anxious about leaving your baby.

Balancing motherhood and a career is a journey that requires planning, flexibility, and a lot of self-compassion. Let's explore some tips to help you navigate this new chapter with confidence and grace.

Preparing for Your Return

Before your first day back, take some steps to prepare both practically and emotionally:

Plan Ahead: Start planning your return a few weeks in advance. Arrange childcare, familiarize yourself with any new routines, and consider a trial run to ease the transition.

Communicate with Your Employer: Discuss your return date, work schedule, and any necessary adjustments with your employer. Clarify expectations and express any concerns you may have.

Ease Into It: If possible, consider a gradual return to work. Start with part-time hours or a flexible schedule to help you and your baby adjust.

Choosing the Right Childcare

Finding reliable and nurturing childcare is crucial for your peace of mind:

Research Options: Explore different childcare options such as daycare centers, nannies, or family members. Visit facilities, check references, and ask about their policies and routines.

Trust Your Instincts: Choose a childcare provider that feels right for you and your baby. Trusting your caregiver will help you feel more at ease when you're at work.

Prepare Your Baby: Gradually introduce your baby to their new caregiver or environment. Spend time together during the first few days to help them adjust.

Managing Your Time

Balancing work and motherhood requires effective time management and flexibility:

Create a Schedule: Develop a daily schedule that balances work commitments, childcare, and family time. Include time for self-care and relaxation.

Prioritize Tasks: Focus on essential tasks and delegate when possible. Let go of the need for perfection and accept help from others.

Stay Organized: Use calendars, to-do lists, and apps to keep track of appointments, deadlines, and family activities.

Maintaining a strong bond with your baby while working is important for both of you:

Quality Time: Make the most of the time you have with your baby. Focus on quality interactions, such as reading, playing, and cuddling.

Stay in Touch: Check in with your caregiver during the day for updates and photos. This can help you feel more connected and reassured.

Special Rituals: Create special routines for mornings and evenings, like a morning snuggle or a bedtime story, to maintain a sense of closeness.

Finding Support

Seeking support from others can make the transition smoother:

Partner Support: Communicate openly with your partner about your feelings and responsibilities. Share household and childcare duties to lighten the load.

Workplace Support: Reach out to colleagues or other working parents for advice and support. Some workplaces have parent support groups or networks.

Professional Help: If you're struggling with the transition, consider speaking to a counselor or therapist who specializes in postpartum or working-parent issues.

Embracing Flexibility

Remember that balancing work and motherhood is an evolving process:

Adjust as Needed: Be prepared to adjust your routines and expectations as you and your baby grow and change. Flexibility is key to finding balance.

Celebrate Achievements: Acknowledge and celebrate your successes, no matter how small. You're doing a remarkable job managing both roles.

Give Yourself Grace: Be kind to yourself on tough days. It's normal to feel overwhelmed at times, and it's okay to ask for help or take a break.

Returning to work while balancing motherhood is a significant and sometimes challenging transition.

By planning ahead, staying organized, and seeking support, you can navigate this journey with confidence.

Remember, it's a balancing act that will require adjustments along the way, and that's perfectly okay.

Maintaining Relationships: Partner, Family, and Friends

Welcoming a baby into your life is an exciting and transformative experience, but it also brings new challenges to your relationships.

Amid the sleepless nights and endless diaper changes, it's important to nurture your connections with your partner, family, and friends.

Strengthening Your Partnership

Your relationship with your partner is the foundation of your family. Here's how to keep it strong:

Communicate Openly: Make time to talk about your feelings, concerns, and joys. Honest communication helps you understand each other's perspectives and needs.

Share Responsibilities: Work together to divide household and baby duties. Sharing the load can prevent resentment and help you feel like a team.

Date Nights: Even if it's just a quiet dinner at home after the baby is asleep, try to carve out regular time for just the two of you. It's important to reconnect as a couple.

Show Appreciation: Small gestures of gratitude and appreciation can go a long way. A simple thank you or a note of encouragement can boost each other's spirits.

Connecting with Family

Your family can be a wonderful source of support and love. Here's how to keep those bonds strong:

Involve Them in Your Baby's Life: Share updates, photos, and milestones with your family. Inviting them to be part of your baby's journey can strengthen your connections.

Ask for Help: Don't hesitate to reach out for help with childcare, meals, or household tasks. Family members are often eager to lend a hand and feel involved.

Set Boundaries: It's okay to set boundaries with family members regarding visits and advice. Clear, respectful communication can help manage expectations and maintain harmony.

Cherish Traditions: Continue or create new family traditions that include your baby. These rituals can provide a sense of continuity and belonging.

Staying Close with Friends

Your friends can provide invaluable emotional support and companionship. Here's how to maintain those friendships:

Stay in Touch: Even if you can't meet in person, stay connected through phone calls, texts, or video chats. Sharing your experiences can keep your friendships strong.

Be Honest: Let your friends know if you're feeling overwhelmed or need support. True friends will understand and be there for you.

Plan Meetups: Arrange playdates, coffee mornings, or outings where you can bring your baby along. This allows you to spend time with friends while caring for your little one.

Make Time for Yourself: When possible, take some time for yourself and meet friends without the baby. It's important to nurture your own identity and enjoy adult company.

Balancing Time and Energy

Finding balance between your relationships and your new responsibilities as a mum can be challenging. Here's how to manage your time and energy:

Prioritize Relationships: Identify which relationships are most important to you and focus your energy there. It's okay to step back from less supportive or demanding relationships.

Be Flexible: Understand that your availability and energy levels will fluctuate. Be flexible with plans and communicate openly if you need to reschedule.

Quality Over Quantity: Focus on the quality of interactions rather than the quantity. Meaningful conversations and time spent together can be more fulfilling than frequent but rushed meetings.

Embracing Change

Accept that relationships will evolve as you navigate this new chapter of life:

Grow Together: Embrace the changes in your relationships as opportunities for growth. Parenthood can deepen your connections and create new shared experiences.

Be Patient: Give yourself and your loved ones time to adjust to the new dynamics. Patience and understanding can help ease the transition.

Celebrate Small Wins: Celebrate the small victories in maintaining your relationships. Every effort you make to connect and support each other is a step towards stronger bonds.

Maintaining relationships while adjusting to life with a new baby can be challenging, but it's also incredibly rewarding. By nurturing your connections with your partner, family, and friends, you create a supportive network that enriches your life and your baby's development.

You're doing an amazing job, mama. Remember that it's okay to ask for help and to take time for the people who matter most to you. Trust yourself, lean on your support system, and enjoy the journey of building a loving and connected family.

You've got this, mama! Embrace the love and support around you, and know that your relationships are an essential part of your beautiful new life.

Conclusion

As you reach the end of this handbook, I hope you feel more empowered, informed, and supported in your journey into motherhood.

From the moment you discovered you were pregnant to preparing for your baby's arrival and navigating those first precious weeks, each step of this journey has been filled with unique challenges and incredible joys.

Reflecting on Your Strength and Resilience

Take a moment to reflect on your strength and resilience. Pregnancy, childbirth, and the early days of motherhood are transformative experiences that require immense courage and adaptability.

You've faced changes, uncertainties, and new responsibilities with grace and determination. Celebrate your achievements, no matter how small they may seem. Each one is a testament to your love and dedication as a mother.

Building Your Support Network

Remember, you are not alone on this journey. Surround yourself with a support network of family, friends, healthcare providers, and fellow mums who can offer guidance, lend a listening ear, and share in your experiences.

Don't hesitate to reach out for help when you need it. Embracing support is a sign of strength, not weakness.

Trusting Your Instincts

Trust your instincts and give yourself grace. You know your baby better than anyone else, and your intuition is a powerful tool in nurturing and caring for your little one.

There will be moments of doubt and uncertainty, but always remember that you are doing your best, and that is more than enough.

Embracing the Journey Ahead

Motherhood is a continuous journey of learning and growth. There will be highs and lows, moments of joy and exhaustion, but through it all, you will continue to grow into the amazing mother you are meant to be. Embrace each stage, cherish the little moments, and take things one day at a time.

Self-Care and Well-Being

Taking care of yourself is just as important as taking care of your baby. Prioritize self-care, whether it's through rest, hobbies, exercise, or simply finding moments of peace amidst the chaos. Your well-being is essential for your own happiness and for providing the best care for your baby.

Celebrating the Love and Joy

Finally, celebrate the love and joy that motherhood brings. The bond you share with your baby is like no other, and the love you give and receive will shape your family's future. Treasure these moments, for they are the foundation of a lifetime of memories.

Thank you for allowing me to be a part of your journey into motherhood. I hope this handbook has provided you with valuable insights, practical advice, and heartfelt encouragement.

You are an incredible mother, and your journey is uniquely your own. Embrace it with an open heart, and know that you have everything you need to thrive.

You've got this, mama! Wishing you all the love, joy, and strength as you continue your beautiful adventure in motherhood.